Plant-Based dessert&drink

Super tasty recipes of Plant-Based drinks and dessert to eat healthily and stay fit!

Carolyn J. Perez

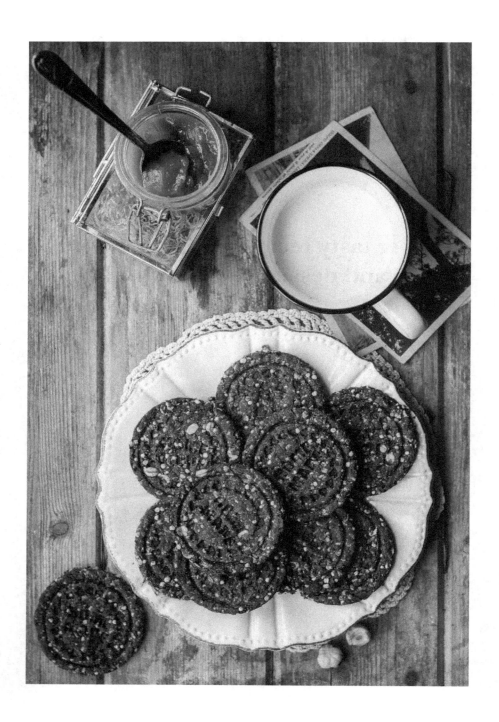

Contents

Introduction

It is a common thought to think that following a diet is necessarily linked to the concept of actual weight loss. However, this is not always the case: following a diet is often directly linked to the foods that we decide to include in our tables daily.

In addition, we do not always choose the best quality ingredients to cook our dishes.

Sometimes we are so rushed and unruly that we forget that we love our bodies. And what better cure than a healthy diet? Following a healthy diet should become more than an imposition or a punishment, but a real lifestyle.

Moreover, this is the Plant-based diet goal: not to impose a restrictive and sometimes impossible diet to follow, but to recreate a diet based on foods of natural origin and above all healthy. Therefore, the plant based represents a real food trend. However, as we will see it is much more than just a fashion trend, but a real lifestyle.

In addition, it is the aim of this text, or rather of this cookbook, to introduce you to the plant based discipline. And we will do it with a few theoretical explanations, just to make you understand what we are talking about and above all how to prepare it: there will be a purely practical part where you will find 50 recipes on the plant based. These recipes will be divided into appetizers, snacks, first and second courses, side dishes and finally a string of plant based desserts.

In the end, you will be spoiled for choice to start following this healthy dietary discipline.

Plant based diet: what are we talking about?

We already mentioned that more than a real weight loss diet the Plant based diet is a food discipline. Food discipline is enjoying great success not only because it is very fashionable, but because it applies such principles that can be perfectly integrated into our daily lives. The plant-based diet is a true approach to life, starting with nutrition: respect for one's health and body, first of all, which is reflected in respect for all forms of life and the planet in general.

As the word itself says, it deals with a food plan based, precisely on what comes from plants. However, simply calling it that way would be too simplistic.

It is a predominantly plant-based diet, but not only. It is not just about consuming vegetables but about taking natural foods: not industrially processed, not treated, and not deriving from the exploitation of resources and animals, preferably zero km.

So it could be a discipline that aims not only at environmental saving but also at the economic one: think about what advantages, in fact, at the level of your pockets you can have if you apply the principle of 0Km and therefore to be able to harvest your vegetables directly from your garden.

Environmental savings do not only mean pollution reduction: the ethical component (present exclusively in the vegan diet, for example) is combined with a strong will to health. This means that the plant based, in addition to not preferring foods that exploit animals, is also based on foods that are especially unprocessed, fresh, healthy, balanced, light, and rich in essential nutrients. In practice, it is a plant-based diet but not vegan / vegetarian, emphasizing the quality and wholesomeness of foods rather than on their moral value, albeit with great attention to sustainability. Such a lifestyle could therefore be of help, not only to our health, but also to create a more sustainable world for future generations.

Main differences between Vegan and Plant based diet

The plant-based diet is often associated with the vegan diet. This is because both plan to include cruelty free foods that do not involve any animal exploitation.

Furthermore, they are associated precisely because they are both predominantly plant-based.

However, there are some pretty obvious differences between these two diets.

First of all, precisely for the reasoning behind the prevalence of plants.

It is well known that even the vegan diet provides a diet based on foods of plant origin: unlike the plant-based diet, however, nothing of animal derivation is allowed, neither direct nor indirect, nor other products - clothing or accessories - which include the exploitation of animals.

No eggs, no milk, no honey, no leather, so to speak, and not only: in its most rigorous meanings, veganism does not even include the use of yeasts, as the bacteria that compose them are indisputably living beings.

A vegan diet can be balanced if the person who leads it knows well the foods and their combinations, the necessary supplements, and their body's reaction to the lack of certain foods.

On the contrary, the Plant-Based diet is on the one hand more relaxed, on the other more stringent.

What does it mean?

This means that it is on the one hand more relaxed because it is plant-based, but not exclusively vegetable: products of animal origin are allowed, in moderate quantities, but under only one condition, namely the excellent quality of the food itself and its certified origin. For example, eggs can be consumed occasionally but only if very fresh, possibly at zero km, from free-range farms where the hens are not exploited but can live outdoors without constraints.

It is also a somewhat more stringent philosophy than veganism precisely for this reason: as long as it is 100% vegetable, the vegan also consumes heavily processed foods, such as industrial fries. Therefore, the vegan can also eat junk foods or snacks. Conversely, plant-based dieters would never admit highly refined foods of this type.

Both dietary approaches are conscious and do not involve the consumption of meat. However, if vegans are driven by ethical reasons, those who follow a plant-based diet also reject everything processed on an industrial level and unhealthy.

A plant-based diet is a diet that aims to eliminate industrially processed foods and, therefore, potentially more harmful to health. It is based on the consumption of fruit and vegetables, whole grains and avoiding (or minimizing) animal products and processed foods. This means that vegan desserts made with refined sugar or bleached flour are also covered.

There is also a substantial difference between the philosophies behind the two diets. As we said in the previous paragraph and above, the ethical component, which is based on the refusal of any food of animal origin, plays a lot in veganism. While for the plant based is not a purely moral and moralistic discourse but on the real thought of being able to keep healthy with the food discipline and be respectful of the environment surrounding us.

Plant based diet full shopping list. What to eat and what to avoid

Now we can examine the complete shopping list of the plant based diet.
Let's briefly summarize the principles on which this particular type of diet is based:

- Emphasizes whole, minimally processed foods.
- Limits or avoids animal products.
- Focuses on plants, including vegetables, fruits, whole grains, legumes, seeds and nuts, which should make up most of what you eat.
- Excludes refined foods, like added sugars, white flour and processed oils.
- Pays special attention to food quality, promoting locally sourced, organic food whenever possible.

As for what you can usually eat, we can say the general consumption of:

- Wholegrain and flours
- extra virgin olive oil

- Seasonal fruit and vegetables: these foods are the basis of every meal.

- In this diet you can also eat sweets but only and exclusively homemade and with controlled raw materials, simple and not very refined, preferably of vegetable origin - for example by replacing milk with soy or rice drinks, and eggs with other natural thickeners such as flaxseed, or simple ripe banana.

- You can also consume nuts and seeds.

As for absolutely forbidden foods, there are all those ready-made and processed:

- ready-made sauces
- chips
- biscuits
- various kinds of snacks
- sugary cereals,
- Spreads, snacks and many other notoriously unhealthy foods.
- Junk food and fast food are therefore absolutely banned
- Sugar beverages

Regarding the complete shopping list:

- Fruits: Berries, citrus fruits, pears, peaches, pineapple, bananas, etc.

- Vegetables: Kale, spinach, tomatoes, broccoli, cauliflower, carrots, asparagus, peppers, etc.

- Starchy vegetables: Potatoes, sweet potatoes, butternut squash, etc.

- Whole grains: Brown rice, rolled oats, spelt, quinoa, brown rice pasta, barley, etc.

- Healthy fats with omega 3: Avocados, olive oil, coconut oil, unsweetened coconut, etc.

- Legumes: Peas, chickpeas, lentils, peanuts, beans, black beans, etc.

- Seeds, nuts and nut butter: Almonds, cashews, macadamia nuts, pumpkin seeds, sunflower seeds, natural peanut butter, tahini, etc.

- Unsweetened plant-based milk: Coconut milk, almond milk, cashew milk, etc.

- Spices, herbs and seasonings: Basil, rosemary, turmeric, curry, black pepper, salt, etc.

- Condiments: Salsa, mustard, nutritional yeast, soy sauce, vinegar, lemon juice, etc.

- Plant-based protein: Tofu, tempeh, seitan, and plant based protein sources or powders with no added sugar or artificial ingredients.
- Beverages: Coffee, tea, sparkling water, etc.

There is the chance to add food of animal origin very rarely, for example if you have specific nutritional needs or if it has been strongly recommended by your doctor. Anyway, if supplementing your plant-based diet with animal products choose quality products from grocery stores or, better yet, purchase them from local farms.

- Eggs: Pasture-raised when possible.
- Poultry: Free-range, organic when possible.
- Beef and pork: Pastured or grass-fed when possible.
- Seafood: Wild-caught from sustainable fisheries when possible.
- Dairy: Organic dairy products from pasture-raised animals whenever possible.

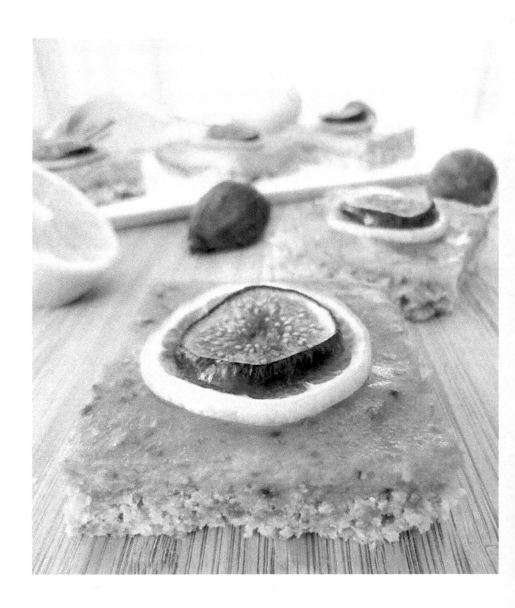

Dessert and fruit recipes

Coconut and walnuts truffles

PREARATION TIME: 20 minutes
COOK TIME: 15 minutes
CALORIES: 300

INGREDIENTS FOR 5/6 SERVINGS
- 50 grams of coconut oil

- 50 grams coconut flour (dehydrated coconut)

- 50 grams of almond flour

- 50 grams of walnut kernels

- 50 grams of vegan brown sugar

- Coconut flour to taste

DIRECTIONS

1. Let us start recipe by melting coconut oil in the microwave.

2. Then take the walnut kernels and chop them finely

3. In a rather large bowl, combine the coconut flour, almond flour, brown sugar and chopped walnuts with the coconut oil.

4. The size of the bowl will allow you to work more easily by having to draw directly with your hands to make the balls.

5. Now, mix well making sure you get a homogeneous mixture.

6. Lightly moisten your hands and form small balls slightly smaller than a walnut with the dough.

7. Moistening your hands is a little trick to keep them from sticking.

8. When the truffles are ready, line them up on the baking tray.

9. Bake them in the oven for 14/15 minutes or until they are slightly golden.

10. Let them cool. Sprinkle with coconut flour.

11. Now, truffles are ready to be served.

Plums jam and almond tart

PREPARATION TIME: 75 minutes
COOKING TIME: 150 minutes
CALORIES: 480

INGREDIENTS FOR 6/8 SERVINGS

- 150 grams' wholemeal flour

- 100 grams' almond flour

- 80 grams of corn oil

- 60 ml of water

- 8 grams of natural yeast based on cream of tartar

- zest of 1/2 lemon

- 120 g of vegan whole cane sugar

- 500 grams of homemade plum jam (see recipe)

- 40 grams of chopped almonds

DIRECTIONS

1. Start with the pastry preparation.

2. In a large bowl put all the dry ingredients and sift them to avoid lumps.

3. This step will make cooking easier and make the mixture more digestible. Blend the brown sugar in a blender equipped with blades in order to pulverize it and avoid leaving grains inside the shortcrust pastry.

4. Add the brown sugar and grated lemon zest to the flour. Add the powders to the liquids and mix well, until the mixture is workable with

your hands. Transfer the mixture to a work surface, preferably a wooden one, and knead until a homogeneous dough is obtained.

5. Wrap the dough in cling film and let it rest in the refrigerator for at least 1 hour.

6. Once the rest period has passed, roll out the pastry on a work surface and then place it in the pan: it is a very crumbly pastry, so while you roll it out, be delicate.

7. Prick the bottom with the tines of a fork. With the leftover dough, make shapes to decorate the tart.

8. Now pour the plums jam into the raw shortcrust pastry.

9. Sprinkle over chopped almonds, shell and cook for 30/40 minutes at 180 C °, static oven.

10. Serve the tarts when it has cooled down.

Rhubarb apples and cinnamon compote tart

PREPARATION TIME: 75 minutes
COOKING TIME: 150 minutes
CALORIES: 492

INGREDIENTS FOR 6/8 SERVINGS

- 150 grams wholemeal flour
- 100 grams almond flour
- 80 grams of corn oil
- 60 ml of water
- 8 grams of natural yeast based on cream of tartar
- zest of 1/2 lemon
- 120 g of vegan whole cane sugar
- 500 grams of rhubarb apples and cinnamon compote (see recipe)

DIRECTIONS

1. Start with the pastry preparation.
2. In a large bowl put all the dry ingredients and sift them to avoid lumps.
3. This step will make cooking easier and make the mixture more digestible. Blend the brown sugar in a blender equipped with blades in order to pulverize it and avoid leaving grains inside the shortcrust pastry.
4. Add the brown sugar and grated lemon zest to the flour. Add the powders to the liquids and mix well, until the mixture is workable with your hands. Transfer the mixture to a work surface, preferably a wooden one, and knead until a homogeneous dough is obtained.

5. Wrap the dough in cling film and let it rest in the refrigerator for at least 1 hour.

6. Once the rest period has passed, roll out the pastry on a work surface and then place it in the pan: it is a very crumbly pastry, so while you roll it out, be delicate.

7. Prick the bottom with the tines of a fork. With the leftover dough, make shapes to decorate the tart.

8. Now pour rhubarb apples and cinnamon compote into the raw shortcrust pastry.

9. Shell and cook for 30/40 minutes at 180 C °, static oven.

10. Serve the tarts when it has cooled down.

Rolled oats and blueberries tart

PREPARATION TIME: 15 minutes
REST TIME: 20 minutes
COOKING TIME: 50 minutes
CALORIES: 390

INGREDIENTS FOR 8/10 SERVINGS

- 350 grams of rolled oats
- 130 grams vegan raw cane sugar
- 80 grams cold water
- 65 ml sunflower oil
- ½ lemon zest and juice
- 5 ml of vanilla extract
- 1 pinch of salt
- 12 grams baking powder
- 500 grams of fresh blueberries
- 3 tablespoons of vegan brown sugar

DIRECTIONS

1. Blend the oat flakes in a blender until you get a fine flour and set aside.
2. Take the fresh blueberries and add them to a bowl with 3 tablespoons of sugar and the juice of half a lemon.
3. Stir and set aside to marinate.
4. In a large bowl pour the sunflower oil, water, sugar, lemon zest, vanilla extract and mix well with a spatula until the sugar has dissolved.

5. Add the oatmeal (or any other flour of your choice), salt and baking powder all at once and mix again.

6. When the dough is firm enough, start kneading with your hands for a minute to better combine the ingredients, not kneading excessively.

7. Let the dough rest in the refrigerator for about 20 minutes, putting it back in the bowl covered with a kitchen towel.

8. Now prepare the pan by greasing it with a little oil, then dusted with flour.

9. Preheat the oven to 180º C.

10. Take about ¾ of the dough and shape it into a ball shape, then slowly flatten it with a rolling pin until you get a thickness of about 4-5 mm.

11. Roll the dough around the rolling pin to lift it and place it in the pan, cutting off the excess. With a fork, make holes in the dough.

12. Add the fresh blueberries and spread them on the pan.

13. Take the rest of the dough (you should have about ¼) and roll it out in a rectangular on the table. Then, with a sharp knife, cut 9 or 10 strips about 1 cm wide.

14. Place the first 5 strips on the cake at the same distance from each other, and then place the other 4 or 5 strips on top, but diagonally.

15. Once this is done, seal the cake by pressing with your fingers where the strips meet the edge of the base. Brush the top of the tart with water or vegetable milk.

16. cover the tart with dough strips

17. Bake in the oven at 180 °C for about 40 minutes.

18. The cake is ready when you see it is golden.

19. Remove from the oven, let cool and serve.

Rolled oats and Nutella tart

PREPARATION TIME: 15 minutes
REST TIME: 20 minutes
COOKING TIME: 50 minutes
CALORIES: 485

INGREDIENTS FOR 8/10 SERVINGS

- 350 grams of rolled oats

- 130 grams vegan raw cane sugar

- 80 grams cold water

- 65 ml sunflower oil

- ½ lemon zest and juice

- 5 ml of vanilla extract

- 1 pinch of salt

- 12 grams baking powder

- 400 grams of Nutella homemade cream (see basic recipe)

DIRECTIONS

1. Blend the oat flakes in a blender until you get a fine flour and set aside.

2. In a large bowl pour the sunflower oil, water, sugar, lemon zest, vanilla extract and mix well with a spatula until the sugar has dissolved.

3. Add the oatmeal (or any other flour of your choice), salt and baking powder all at once and mix again.

4. When the dough is firm enough, start kneading with your hands for a minute to better combine the ingredients, not kneading excessively.

5. Let the dough rest in the refrigerator for about 20 minutes, putting it back in the bowl covered with a kitchen towel.

6. Now prepare the pan by greasing it with a little oil, then dusted with flour.

7. Preheat the oven to 180º C.

8. Take about ¾ of the dough and shape it into a ball shape, then slowly flatten it with a rolling pin until you get a thickness of about 4-5 mm.

9. Roll the dough around the rolling pin to lift it and place it in the pan, cutting off the excess. With a fork, make holes in the dough.

10. Add the Nutella cream and spread them on the pan.

11. Take the rest of the dough (you should have about ¼) and roll it out in a rectangular on the table. Then, with a sharp knife, cut 9 or 10 strips about 1 cm wide.

12. Place the first 5 strips on the cake at the same distance from each other, and then place the other 4 or 5 strips on top, but diagonally.

13. Once this is done, seal the cake by pressing with your fingers where the strips meet the edge of the base. Brush the top of the tart with water or vegetable milk.

14. cover the tart with dough strips

15. Bake in the oven at 180 °C for about 40 minutes.

16. The cake is ready when you see it is golden.

17. Remove from the oven, let cool and serve.

Oat and vanilla custard tart

PREPARATION TIME: 15 minutes
REST TIME: 20 minutes
COOKING TIME: 50 minutes
CALORIES: 460

INGREDIENTS FOR 8/10 SERVINGS

- 350 grams of rolled oats
- 130 grams vegan raw cane sugar
- 80 grams cold water
- 65 ml sunflower oil
- ½ lemon zest and juice
- 5 ml of vanilla extract
- 1 pinch of salt
- 12 grams baking powder
- 500 grams of vanilla homemade custard (see basic recipe)

DIRECTIONS

1. Blend the oat flakes in a blender until you get a fine flour and set aside.
2. In a large bowl pour the sunflower oil, water, sugar, lemon zest, vanilla extract and mix well with a spatula until the sugar has dissolved.
3. Add the oatmeal (or any other flour of your choice), salt and baking powder all at once and mix again.
4. When the dough is firm enough, start kneading with your hands for a minute to better combine the ingredients, not kneading excessively.

5. Let the dough rest in the refrigerator for about 20 minutes, putting it back in the bowl covered with a kitchen towel.

6. Now prepare the pan by greasing it with a little oil, then dusted with flour.

7. Preheat the oven to 180º C.

8. Take about ¾ of the dough and shape it into a ball shape, then slowly flatten it with a rolling pin until you get a thickness of about 4-5 mm.

9. Roll the dough around the rolling pin to lift it and place it in the pan, cutting off the excess. With a fork, make holes in the dough.

10. Add the vanilla custard and spread them on the pan.

11. Take the rest of the dough (you should have about ¼) and roll it out in a rectangular shape on the table. Then, with a sharp knife, cut 9 or 10 strips about 1 cm wide.

12. Place the first 5 strips on the cake at the same distance from each other, and then place the other 4 or 5 strips on top, but diagonally.

13. Once this is done, seal the cake by pressing with your fingers where the strips meet the edge of the base. Brush the top of the tart with water or vegetable milk.

14. cover the tart with dough strips

15. Bake in the oven at 180 °C for about 40 minutes.

16. The cake is ready when you see it is golden.

17. Remove from the oven, let cool and serve.

Oat and pistachio custard tart

PREPARATION TIME: 15 minutes
REST TIME: 20 minutes
COOKING TIME: 50 minutes
CALORIES: 502

INGREDIENTS FOR 8/10 SERVINGS

- 350 grams of rolled oats
- 130 grams vegan raw cane sugar
- 80 grams cold water
- 65 ml sunflower oil
- ½ lemon zest and juice
- 5 ml of vanilla extract
- 1 pinch of salt
- 12 grams baking powder
- 500 grams of pistachio homemade custard (see basic recipe)

DIRECTIONS

1. Blend the oat flakes in a blender until you get a fine flour and set aside.
2. In a large bowl pour the sunflower oil, water, sugar, lemon zest, vanilla extract and mix well with a spatula until the sugar has dissolved.
3. Add the oatmeal (or any other flour of your choice), salt and baking powder all at once and mix again.
4. When the dough is firm enough, start kneading with your hands for a minute to better combine the ingredients, not kneading excessively.

5. Let the dough rest in the refrigerator for about 20 minutes, putting it back in the bowl covered with a kitchen towel.
6. Now prepare the pan by greasing it with a little oil, then dusted with flour.
7. Preheat the oven to 180º C.
8. Take about ¾ of the dough and shape it into a ball shape, then slowly flatten it with a rolling pin until you get a thickness of about 4-5 mm.
9. Roll the dough around the rolling pin to lift it and place it in the pan, cutting off the excess. With a fork, make holes in the dough.
10. Add the pistachio custard and spread them on the pan.
11. Take the rest of the dough (you should have about ¼) and roll it out in a rectangular shape on the table. Then, with a sharp knife, cut 9 or 10 strips about 1 cm wide.
12. Place the first 5 strips on the cake at the same distance from each other, and then place the other 4 or 5 strips on top, but diagonally.
13. Once this is done, seal the cake by pressing with your fingers where the strips meet the edge of the base. Brush the top of the tart with water or vegetable milk.
14. cover the tart with dough strips
15. Bake in the oven at 180 °C for about 40 minutes.
16. The cake is ready when you see it is golden.
17. Remove from the oven, let cool and serve.

Apple and figs tart

PREPARATION TIME: 20 minutes
REST TIME: 1 hour in the fridge
COOKING TIME: 150 minutes
CALORIES: 460

INGREDIENTS FOR 10 SERVINGS

For the tart:
- 500 grams wholemeal flour
- 125 grams wholemeal spelt flour
- 150 grams brown rice syrup
- 100 grams maple syrup
- 125 grams sunflower oil
- 3 teaspoons of cream of tartar (or natural yeast powder)
- a pinch of vanilla powder
- 1 pinch of salt
- 120 ml of water

For the apple and figs filling:
- 100 grams of vegan brown sugar
- 3 golden apples
- 500 grams of figs
- 2 tablespoons of water
- cinnamon to taste
- 1 lime (zest and juice)

DIRECTIONS

1. In a large bowl, combine all the dry ingredients, then the wholemeal flours, the spelt one, yeast, vanilla and salt.

2. Separately, mix the oil, syrups and water, which you will then add to the dry ingredients.

3. Mix everything well and knead the dough for a few minutes.

4. At the end, you will have to obtain a homogeneous dough that you will leave to rest in the refrigerator wrapped in cling film for half an hour.

5. Meanwhile, you can prepare filling.

6. Peel the apples by removing the skins and cut them into cubes about one centimetre thick.

7. To prevent the apples from oxidizing while you are cutting them all, place them in a bowl with water and juice of half a lemon.

8. After the apples, pass the figs, clean them and cut them into wedges.

9. In a non-stick pan, heat the sugar and add the water: cook over low heat until you get a dark brown caramel with a good density, stirring constantly.

10. Now add the apples, figs, cinnamon, grated lime zest, and cook for a few minutes until the apples are well coloured but still crunchy and let cool.

11. Line the pan with parchment paper and divide the dough into these doses: 2/3 for the base of the cake and the rest for the strips to put on top.

12. With a rolling pin, roll out the pastry trying to make a round shape with a thickness of about 5 millimetres and line the pan, including the edges.

13. Then spread the filling of apples and figs with cinnamon and then pass to form strips (or lozenges).

14. Roll out the remaining pastry forming a rectangle and with a toothed wheel or a knife with a thin and smooth blade, make 6 strips about 2 and a half centimetres wide that are a little longer than the diameter of the mold.

15. Arrange 3 strips on the tart parallel to each other, and fold the odd strips in half, perpendicular, arrange the central strip and put back in place.

16. Fold the even strips and do the same operation placing the strip always perpendicularly. You should therefore intertwine the lozenges together.

17. Remove the excess lozenge dough and lightly crush them to make them adhere to the edge of the tart and brush the surface of the cake with a mixture of malt or syrup and water to brown it, then cook in the lower part of the oven (static) at 180 ° for 40 -50 minutes.

18. Remove from the oven and allow cooling to room temperature before serving.

Peach and raspberries tart

PREPARATION TIME: 20 minutes
REST TIME: 1 hour in the fridge
COOKING TIME: 150 minutes
CALORIES: 460

INGREDIENTS FOR 10 SERVINGS

For the tart:
- 500 grams wholemeal flour
- 125 grams wholemeal spelt flour
- 150 grams brown rice syrup
- 100 grams maple syrup
- 125 grams sunflower oil
- 3 teaspoons of cream of tartar (or natural yeast powder)
- a pinch of vanilla powder
- 1 pinch of salt
- 120 ml of water

For the peach and raspberries filling:
- 100 grams of vegan brown sugar
- 3 peaches
- 500 grams of raspberries
- 2 tablespoons of water
- 1 pinch of vanilla powder
- 1 orange (zest and juice)

DIRECTIONS

1. In a large bowl, combine all the dry ingredients, then the wholemeal flours, the spelt one, yeast, vanilla and salt.
2. Separately, mix the oil, syrups and water, which you will then add to the dry ingredients.
3. Mix everything well and knead the dough for a few minutes.
4. At the end, you will have to obtain a homogeneous dough that you will leave to rest in the refrigerator wrapped in cling film for half an hour.
5. Meanwhile, you can prepare filling.
6. Peel the peaches by removing the skins and cut them into cubes about one centimetre thick.
7. After that, clean raspberries them and cut them into pieces.
8. In a non-stick pan, heat the sugar and add the water: cook over low heat until you get a dark brown caramel with a good density, stirring constantly.
9. Now add the peaches, raspberries, vanilla powder, grated orange zest, and juice and cook for a few minutes until the apples are well coloured but still crunchy and let cool.
10. Line the pan with parchment paper and divide the dough into these doses: 2/3 for the base of the cake and the rest for the strips to put on top.
11. With a rolling pin, roll out the pastry trying to make a round shape with a thickness of about 5 millimetres and line the pan, including the edges.
12. Then spread the fruit filling and then pass to form strips (or lozenges).
13. Roll out the remaining pastry forming a rectangle and with a toothed wheel or a knife with a thin and smooth blade, make 6 strips about 2 and a half centimetres wide that are a little longer than the diameter of the mold.

14. Arrange 3 strips on the tart parallel to each other, and fold the odd strips in half, perpendicular, arrange the central strip and put back in place.

15. Fold the even strips and do the same operation placing the strip always perpendicularly. You should therefore intertwine the lozenges together.

16. Remove the excess lozenge dough and lightly crush them to make them adhere to the edge of the tart and brush the surface of the cake with a mixture of malt or syrup and water to brown it, then cook in the lower part of the oven (static) at 180 ° for 40 -50 minutes.

17. Remove from the oven and allow cooling to room temperature before serving.

Apple and almond cream little tart

PREPARATION TIME: 20 minutes
REST TIME: at least 1 hour in the fridge
COOKING TIME: 150 minutes
CALORIES: 485

INGREDIENTS FOR 6/8 SERVINGS

For the tart:
- 160 grams of wholemeal flour
- 40 grams of wholemeal spelt flour
- 100 ml of brown rice syrup
- 55 g sunflower oil
- 1 pinch of salt
- 1 pinch of yeast (cream of tartar)
- ½ teaspoon of vanilla essence (or the seeds of the berry)

For the cream:
- 2–3 red apples
- 200 ml soymilk
- 15 grams of corn starch
- 1 tablespoon of brown rice syrup
- 1 pinch of cinnamon
- ½ teaspoon of vanilla essence (or the seeds of the berry)
- 130 grams all natural almond cream (see basic recipe)

DIRECTIONS

1. Start with the tart dough

2. In a bowl, sift the flour and yeast, add the salt and add the oil, rice syrup and vanilla essence.

3. Mix well with your hands until you get a homogeneous mixture (if it is too dry, moisten it with a drop of vegetable milk).

4. Wrap the pastry in plastic wrap and let it rest in the refrigerator for an hour.

5. in the meantime, prepare the creamy filling. Dissolve the starch directly in a saucepan with a few tablespoons of soymilk, to dissolve all the lumps well.

6. Then pour in the remaining milk, cinnamon and vanilla essence, and cook everything over low heat and without stopping stirring, until the cream has thickened.

7. At this point, add the almond cream and the spoonful of rice syrup and let it cool down covered with a sheet of cling film in direct contact with the surface of the cream.

8. Now wash the apples well, and, keeping the peel cut them into very thin slices with a mandolin or a sharp knife.

9. Divide the pastry dough into 4 and roll it out with a rolling pin to a thickness of 4-5 mm.

10. Lightly grease the little tart molds, gently lay the spread out pastry and cut out the excess dough that comes out of the edges.

11. Decorate the latter to your liking, for example by making decorative motifs with the tip of a teaspoon, as we did. Pour 2 or 3 spoonful of cream into each tart.

12. Take 5-6 slices of apple and put them in a row, overlapping them halfway.

13. Roll them up rather tightly, being careful not to break them, and as the roses are ready, place them on the custard making them sink a little.

14. Once you have filled all the tartlets with the apple decorations, brush them with 1 tablespoon of rice syrup extended with a tablespoon of water, in order to make the surface shiny.

15. Bake at 180 ° C for 30 minutes in a static oven, until the pastry is cooked and golden.

16. Let the tarts cool completely before gently removing them from the molds.

Almond cream and pistachio little tart

PREPARATION TIME: 20 minutes
REST TIME: at least 1 hour in the fridge
COOKING TIME: 150 minutes
CALORIES: 510

INGREDIENTS FOR 6/8 SERVINGS

For the tart:
- 160 grams of wholemeal flour

- 40 grams of almond flour

- 100 grams of brown rice syrup

- 55 ml of sunflower oil

- 1 pinch of salt

- 1 pinch of yeast (cream of tartar)

- ½ teaspoon of vanilla essence (or the seeds of the berry)

For the cream:
- 100 grams of chopped pistachios

- 200 ml soymilk

- 15 grams of corn starch

- 1 tablespoon of brown rice syrup

- 1 pinch of cinnamon

- ½ teaspoon of vanilla essence

- 150 grams all natural almond cream (see basic recipe)

DIRECTIONS

1. Start with the tart dough

2. In a bowl, sift the two flour and yeast, add the salt and add the oil, rice syrup and vanilla essence.

3. Mix well with your hands until you get a homogeneous mixture (if it is too dry, moisten it with a drop of vegetable milk).

4. Wrap the pastry in plastic wrap and let it rest in the refrigerator for an hour.

5. in the meantime, prepare the creamy filling. Dissolve the starch directly in a saucepan with a few tablespoons of soymilk, so as to dissolve all the lumps well.

6. Then pour in the remaining milk, cinnamon and vanilla essence, and cook everything over low heat and without stopping stirring, until the cream has thickened.

7. At this point, add the almond cream the chopped pistachios, and the spoonful of rice syrup and let it cool down covered with a sheet of cling film in direct contact with the surface of the cream.

8. Divide the pastry dough into 4 and roll it out with a rolling pin to a thickness of 4-5 mm.

9. Lightly grease the little tart molds, gently lay the spread out pastry and cut out the excess dough that comes out of the edges.

10. Decorate the latter to your liking, for example by making decorative motifs with the tip of a teaspoon, as we did. Pour 2 or 3 spoonful of cream into each tart.

11. Take 5-6 slices of apple and put them in a row, overlapping them halfway.

12. Roll them up rather tightly, being careful not to break them, and as the roses are ready, place them on the custard making them sink a little.

13. Once you have filled all the tartlets with the apple decorations, brush them with 1 tablespoon of rice syrup extended with a tablespoon of water, in order to make the surface shiny.

14. Bake at 180° C for 30 minutes in a static oven, until the pastry is cooked and golden.

15. Let the tarts cool completely before gently removing them from the molds.

Apple and dried fruits strudel

PREPARATION TIME: 40 minutes
COOKING TIME: 30 minutes
CALORIES: 390

INGREDIENTS FOR 6/8 SERVINGS

For the pastry:
- 100 grams of rice flour
- 100 grams of soy flour
- 35 grams of corn starch
- 5 g of guar gum (or xanthan or tara gum)
- 90 grams of vegan brown sugar
- 160 ml of soymilk

For the apple and dried fruits stuffing:
- 2 apples
- 20 grams of vegan brown sugar
- 10 blueberries
- 1 pinch of powdered ginger
- 1 pinch of cinnamon powder
- 2 tablespoons of chopped almonds and pistachios

DIRECTIONS

1. Start the recipe by preparing the strudel dough.
2. Sift the flours, corn starch and guar gum into a bowl.
3. Add the brown sugar and mix the dry ingredients.

4. Slowly add the soymilk until you get a dough that you will go to work for at least ten minutes. You will need to reach a soft and slightly elastic consistency.

5. Now you can move on to prepare the filling.

6. Wash and peel the apples and cut them into cubes.

7. Wash the blueberries too.

8. Peel and chop both pistachios and almonds.

9. In a bowl combine all the ingredients for the filling, then cover with the spices (ginger and cinnamon) and brown sugar and mix.

10. Let it sit for 5 minutes.

11. Roll out the strudel dough to a thickness of about 3 mm giving it a rectangular shape and place the filling in the centre.

12. Close the edges on themselves turn the dough upside down and brush the surface with a mixture of malt and water.

13. Finally, cut with a knife making small cuts.

14. Bake at 180º C for about 30 minutes.

15. Check the cooking and if necessary cook for another 5 minutes.

16. Let it cool and serve.

Classic apple strudel

PREPARATION TIME: 40 minutes
COOKING TIME: 30 minutes
CALORIES: 390

INGREDIENTS FOR 6/8 SERVINGS

For the pastry:
- 100 grams of rice flour
- 100 grams of soy flour
- 35 grams of corn starch
- 5 g of guar gum (or xanthan or tara gum)
- 90 grams of vegan brown sugar
- 160 ml of soymilk

For the apple filling:
- 2 big apples
- 20 grams of vegan brown sugar
- 1 pinch of powdered ginger
- 1 pinch of cinnamon powder
- 1 pinch of vanilla powder
- 1 tablespoon of marble syrup

DIRECTIONS

1. Start the recipe by preparing the strudel dough.
2. Sift the flours, corn starch and guar gum into a bowl.
3. Add the brown sugar and mix the dry ingredients.

4. Slowly add the soymilk until you get a dough that you will go to work for at least ten minutes. You will need to reach a soft and slightly elastic consistency.

5. Now you can move on to prepare the filling.

6. Wash and peel the apples and cut them into little cubes.

7. In a bowl, combine apple cubes with the spices (ginger, vanilla and cinnamon) marble syrup and brown sugar.

8. Mix well and let it sit for 5 minutes.

9. Roll out the strudel dough to a thickness of about 3 mm giving it a rectangular shape and place the filling in the centre.

10. Close the edges on themselves, turn the dough upside down and brush the surface with a mixture of malt and water.

11. Finally, cut with a knife making small cuts.

12. Bake at 180º C for about 30 minutes.

13. Check the cooking and if necessary cook for another 5 minutes.

14. Let it cool and serve.

Coconut and almonds truffles

PREARATION TIME: 20 minutes
COOK TIME: 15 minutes
CALORIES: 300

INGREDIENTS FOR 5/6 SERVINGS

- 50 grams of almond butter
- 50 grams coconut flour (dehydrated coconut)
- 50 grams of almond flour
- 50 grams of almonds
- 50 grams of vegan brown sugar
- Coconut flour to taste

DIRECTIONS

1. Let us start by melting almond butter in the microwave.
2. Then take the almonds peel and chop them finely
3. In a rather large bowl, combine the coconut flour, almond flour, brown sugar and chopped almonds with almond melted butter.
4. The size of the bowl will allow you to work more easily by having to draw directly with your hands to make the balls.
5. Now, mix well making sure you get a homogeneous mixture.
6. Lightly moisten your hands and form small balls slightly smaller than a walnut with the dough.
7. Moistening your hands is a little trick to keep them from sticking.
8. When the truffles are ready, line them up on the baking tray.

9. Bake them in the oven for 14/15 minutes or until they are slightly golden.

10. Let them cool. Sprinkle with coconut flour.

11. Now, truffles are ready to be served.

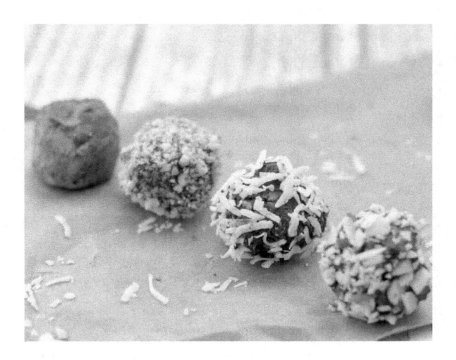

Tofu and chocolate truffles

PREPARATION TIME: 10 minutes
REST TIME: 1 hour in the freezer
CALORIES: 190

INGREDIENTS FOR 4 SERVINGS

- 120 grams of tofu cheese
- 60 grams of softened soy butter
- 50 grams of vegan cane sugar
- 40 grams of almond flour
- 1/4 teaspoon of vanilla extract
- A pinch of salt
- 50 g of vegan dark chocolate chips

DIRECTIONS

1. Start the recipe by beating the tofu cheese and soy butter in a large bowl until well blended.
2. Add the vegan brown sugar, almond flour, vanilla extract, salt, and mix until smooth.
3. Add half of the chocolate chips and stir until well blended.
4. Let the mixture cool in the freezer for about an hour to harden it a little and thus be able to form balls more easily.
5. After the hour, take the dough out of the freezer and, with your hands, form pralines of about 2.5 cm in diameter.
6. If the dough seems too soft, add a little more almond flour.

7. Roll the pralines on a plate where you have put the rest of the chocolate chips, and try to cover them as much as possible with the drops.

8. Serve immediately.

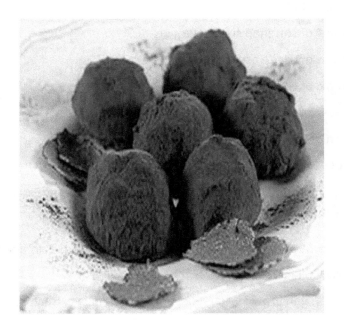

Soy and chocolate truffles

PREPARATION TIME: 10 minutes
REST TIME: 1 hour in the freezer
CALORIES: 205

INGREDIENTS FOR 4 SERVINGS

- 120 grams of soy cheese
- 60 grams of softened soy butter
- 50 grams of vegan cane sugar
- 40 grams of coconut flour
- 1/4 teaspoon of vanilla extract
- A pinch of salt
- 50 g of vegan dark chocolate chips

DIRECTIONS

1. Start the recipe by beating soy cheese and soy butter in a large bowl until well blended.
2. Add the vegan brown sugar, coconut flour, vanilla extract, salt, and mix until smooth.
3. Add half of the chocolate chips and stir until well blended.
4. Let the mixture cool in the freezer for about an hour to harden it a little and thus be able to form balls more easily.
5. After the hour, take the dough out of the freezer and, with your hands, form pralines of about 2.5 cm in diameter.
6. If the dough seems too soft, add a little more coconut flour.

7. Roll the pralines on a plate where you have put the rest of the chocolate chips, and try to cover them as much as possible with the drops.
8. Serve immediate.

Quinoa and chocolate cookies

PREPARATION TIME: 20 minutes
COOKING TIME: 15 minutes
CALORIES: 370

INGREDIENTS FOR 4/5 SERVINGS

- 150 grams of wholemeal flour

- 90 grams of vegan brown sugar

- 10 grams of flaxseed powder

- 60 ml of soymilk

- 40 ml of vegetable oil

- 40 grams of all natural dark chocolate

- 30 grams of puffed quinoa

- 20 grams of corn starch

- 20 grams of sugar free cocoa

- 1 teaspoon of baking powder

- 1 pinch of salt

DIRECTIONS

1. In a large bowl, sift the wholemeal flour, flaxseed powder, corn starch, unsweetened cocoa and baking powder.

2. Then add the brown sugar, puffed quinoa and salt.

3. Stir in order to mix the dry ingredients well together.

4. Finely chop the dark chocolate.

5. Separately, in a bowl or tall glass, mix the oil and soymilk.

6. Now you just have to combine the mixture of the powders and that of the liquids, adding the chopped chocolate.
7. Work the dough first with a fork or wooden spoon and then with your hands.
8. We form the cookies
9. Roll out the dough on a lightly floured surface or between two sheets of parchment paper, until a thickness of 5 millimetres is obtained.
10. With a pastry cutter of the shape you prefer, cut the biscuits and place them on a dripping pan covered with baking paper. Bake in a preheated static oven at 180° C for 15 minutes.
11. Serve cookies warm.

Corn and chocolate cookies

PREPARATION TIME: 20 minutes
COOKING TIME: 15 minutes
CALORIES: 335

INGREDIENTS FOR 4/5 SERVINGS

- 120 grams of wholemeal flour
- 100 grams of corn starch
- 90 grams of vegan brown sugar
- 60 ml of corn milk
- 40 ml of vegetable oil
- 40 grams of all natural dark chocolate
- 20 grams of sugar free cocoa
- 1 teaspoon of baking powder
- 1 pinch of salt

DIRECTIONS

1. In a large bowl, sift the wholemeal flour, corn starch, unsweetened cocoa and baking powder.
2. Then add the brown sugar and salt.
3. Stir in order to mix the dry ingredients well together.
4. Meanwhile, finely chop the dark chocolate.
5. Separately, in a bowl or tall glass, mix the oil and corn milk.
6. Now you just have to combine the mixture of the powders and that of the liquids, adding the chopped chocolate.

7. Work the dough first with a fork or wooden spoon and then with your hands.

8. Roll out the dough on a lightly floured surface or between two sheets of parchment paper, until a thickness of 5 millimetres is obtained.

9. With a pastry cutter of the shape you prefer, cut the biscuits and place them on a dripping pan covered with baking paper. Bake in a preheated static oven at 180° C for 15 minutes.

10. Serve cookies warm.

Flaxseed almond and chocolate cookies

PREPARATION TIME: 15 minutes
COOKING TIME: 10 minutes
CALORIES: 130

INGREDIENTS FOR 4 SERVINGS

- 250 grams of almond flour

- 1 tablespoon of ground flaxseed

- 3 tablespoons water, plus more if necessary

- 2 tablespoons of coconut oil softened but not melted

- 100 grams of vegan brown sugar

- 60 grams of almond butter

- 1 teaspoon of vanilla extract

- 1/2 teaspoon of baking soda

- 1/4 teaspoon of salt

- 70 grams of vegan sugar free chocolate chips

DIRECTIONS

1. First, preheat the oven to 170º C and line a baking sheet with parchment paper.

2. In the bottom of a large bowl, whisk together the ground flaxseed, water, and let thicken for 5 minutes.

3. To the same bowl, add the coconut oil, vegan sugar, almond butter, and vanilla.

4. Whisk until well combined.

5. Add the almond flour and sprinkle the baking soda and salt evenly over the mixture.

6. Use a spatula or wooden spoon to stir until well combined, adding 1 to 2 tablespoons water if the mixture is too dry. Fold in the chocolate chips.

7. Use a 2-tablespoon cookie scoop to scoop the dough onto the baking sheet. Press each ball down slightly and sprinkle with flaky sea salt, if using.

8. Bake for 10 to 13 minutes or until the edges are just starting the brown.

9. Cool on the pan for 5 minutes and then transfer to a wire rack to finish cooling.

10. When the cookies are completely cool, they can be stored in an airtight container or frozen. (To reheat frozen cookies, bake in a 350F oven for 5 minutes or until warmed through.)

Flaxseed pistachios cookies

PREPARATION TIME: 15 minutes
COOKING TIME: 10 minutes
CALORIES: 120

INGREDIENTS FOR 4 SERVINGS

- 230 grams of almond flour
- 1 tablespoon of ground flaxseed
- 2 tablespoon of finely chopped pistachios
- 3 tablespoons water, plus more if necessary
- 2 tablespoons of coconut oil softened but not melted
- 100 grams of vegan brown sugar
- 60 grams of soy butter
- 1 teaspoon of vanilla extract
- 1/2 teaspoon of baking soda
- 1/4 teaspoon of salt

DIRECTIONS

1. First, preheat the oven to 170º C and line a baking sheet with parchment paper.
2. In the bottom of a large bowl, whisk together the ground flaxseed, water, and let thicken for 5 minutes.
3. To the same bowl, add the coconut oil, vegan sugar, soy butter, and vanilla.
4. Whisk until well combined.
5. Meanwhile peel and finely chop pistachios.

6. Add the almond flour, chopped pistachios, and sprinkle the baking soda and salt evenly over the mixture.

7. Use a spatula or wooden spoon to stir until well combined, adding 1 to 2 tablespoons water if the mixture is too dry.

8. Use a 2-tablespoon cookie scoop to scoop the dough onto the baking sheet. Press each ball down slightly and sprinkle with flaky sea salt, if using.

9. Bake for 10 to 13 minutes or until the edges are just starting the brown.

10. Cool on the pan for 5 minutes and then transfer to a wire rack to finish cooling.

11. When the cookies are completely cool, they can be stored in an airtight container or frozen. (To reheat frozen cookies, bake in a 350F oven for 5 minutes or until warmed through.)

Chocolate and coconut cookies

PREPARATION TIME: 10 minutes
COOKING TIME: 10 minutes
CALORIES: 175

INGREDIENTS FOR 4 SERVINGS

- 100 grams of almond flour

- 30 grams of coconut flour

- 60 grams of sugar free cocoa powder

- 1 teaspoon natural baking powder

- 1/4 tsp Salt

- 150 grams of vegan cane sugar

- 100 ml of sunflower oil

- 1 tablespoon of coconut milk

- 2 teaspoons of vanilla powder

DIRECTIONS

1. In a large bowl, mix the almond flour, coconut flour, unsweetened cocoa, baking powder, and salt.

2. In a separate bowl, mix the sunflower oil and vegan brown sugar until light and fluffy.

3. Add the coconut milk and vanilla to the butter mixture and mix well to blend the ingredients well.

4. Pour the mixture of dry ingredients over the liquid batter and mix to make a thick paste.

5. Cover the dough with cling film and put it in the fridge to cool for at least an hour.

6. Once cooled, the dough will be ready to be worked.

7. In the meantime, preheat the oven to 180 ° C.

8. Line two baking sheets with parchment paper.

9. Divide the dough into about 20 piles and, with your hands, form cookies of 3.5 cm in length each.

10. Cover them completely and then place them on the prepared trays.

11. Bake the cookies for about 9 minutes or until they are almost completely dry in the centre

12. serve as soon as they have cooled down

Chocolate almonds and oat cookies

PREPARATION TIME: 10 minutes
COOKING TIME: 10 minutes
CALORIES: 156

INGREDIENTS FOR 4 SERVINGS

- 100 grams of almond flour
- 60 grams of oat flour
- 30 grams of sugar free cocoa powder
- 1 teaspoon natural baking powder
- 1/4 tsp Salt
- 150 grams of vegan cane sugar
- 100 ml of sunflower oil
- 1 tablespoon of oat milk
- 2 teaspoons of vanilla powder

DIRECTIONS

1. In a large bowl, mix the almond flour, oat flour, cocoa powder, baking powder, and salt.

2. In a separate bowl, mix the sunflower oil and vegan brown sugar until light and fluffy.

3. Add the oat milk and vanilla to the butter mixture and mix well to blend the ingredients well.

4. Pour the mixture of dry ingredients over the liquid batter and mix to make a thick paste.

5. Cover the dough with cling film and put it in the fridge to cool for at least an hour.

6. Once cooled, the dough will be ready to be worked.

7. In the meantime, preheat the oven to 180 ° C.

8. Line two baking sheets with parchment paper.

9. Divide the dough into about 20 piles and, with your hands, form cookies of 3.5 cm in length each.

10. Cover them completely and then place them on the prepared trays.

11. Bake the cookies for about 9 minutes or until they are almost completely dry in the centre

12. serve as soon as they have cooled down

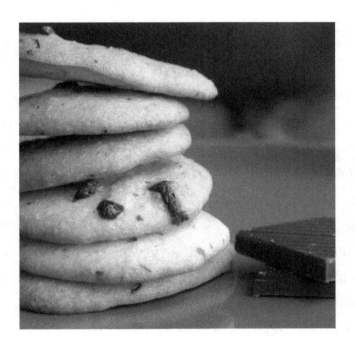

Chocolate and peanut butter cookies

PREPARATION TIME: 20 minutes
REST TIME: 15/20 minutes in the freezer
CALORIES: 205

INGREDIENTS FOR 3/4 SERVINGS

- 70 ml of coconut oil

- 100 grams of peanut butter

- 80 ml of dark maple syrup, divided

- 80 grams of sugar free cocoa powder

- 1 teaspoon of vanilla extract

- 120 grams of rolled oats

- 1 pinch of salt

DIRECTIONS

1. Fist, place 9 cupcake liners into a muffin tin (or 18 liners in a mini-muffin tin).

2. in a small saucepan over low heat, melt 60 ml of coconut oil and stir together 50 grams of peanut butter, 70 ml of cup maple syrup, 70 grams cocoa powder, 1 teaspoon vanilla extract, and 1 pinch of salt.

3. When fully combined, remove from heat and stir in rolled oats. Spoon into cupcake liners. Refrigerate while making the peanut butter topping.

4. In a small saucepan over low heat, stir together the remaining peanut butter, 10 ml of maple syrup, and 10 ml of coconut oil. Spoon the warm peanut butter mixture over the chocolate oat mixture.

5. Freeze for 15 to 20 minutes until set, or refrigerate until serving.

6. Serve cookies cold.

Chocolate frosted almond and peanut butter cookies

PREPARATION TIME: 20 minutes

REST TIME: 25 minutes
COOK TIME: 20/25 minutes
CALORIES: 205

INGREDIENTS FOR 6 SERVINGS

For the almond peanut butter cookies
- 150 grams of wholemeal flour
- 50 grams of almond flour
- 70 ml of coconut oil
- 100 of almond milk
- 1 tablespoon vanilla extract
- 200 grams of creamy peanut butter
- 130 grams of vegan whole cane sugar
- 1/2 teaspoon baking soda
- 1/2 teaspoon baking powder
- 1/2 teaspoon salt

For the vegan chocolate frosting:
- 35 grams of vegan whole cane sugar
- 35 grams of sugar free cocoa powder
- 35 ml of almond milk, plus additional as necessary

DIRECTIONS

1. In a small saucepan over low heat, stir together the coconut oil, milk and vanilla extract until warm and combined.
2. Pour into a large mixing bowl and add the peanut butter and vegan sugar.
3. Stir until well combined (small peanut butter lumps are ok).

4. Add the two flours, baking soda, baking powder and salt and stir with spatula until combined into a cohesive dough.

5. Transfer the dough to a covered container and refrigerate for 25 minutes.

6. Meanwhile, preheat the oven to 180°C.

7. Line two baking sheets with parchment paper.

8. Remove the bowl with the dough from the refrigerator.

9. Make 24 1 1/2 tablespoon-sized balls (using a size 40 cookie scoop, if you have it) and place them onto the baking sheet.

10. Roll the balls between your hands to make them as spherical as possible. Place them 2 inches apart on the baking sheets.

11. Use a fork to flatten the balls and make a criss-cross pattern (it's helpful to dip the fork into a small bowl of water before each one to prevent sticking).

12. Bake each tray separately, about 15 minutes, (rotating halfway through at about 7 minutes) until edges are just firm. Cool for 5 minutes on the tray, and then remove to a cooling rack. (Baking the tray separately gets the most even bake.)

13. Meanwhile, prepare chocolate frosting.

14. In a medium bowl, use a fork to stir together the powdered sugar, cocoa powder and almond milk until a smooth sauce forms and all lumps are dissolved.

15. Add almond milk a teaspoon at a time if necessary until a thick but drizzle-able consistency is reached (be careful not to add too much liquid). Dip a fork into the glaze and drizzle in a zigzag pattern. Let sit at room temperature until the glaze is dry, about 20 to 30 minutes

16. When cookies are ready, serve once cooled to room temperature, with a topping of chocolate frosting.

Black grape and cinnamon cookies

PREPARATION TIME: 20 minutes
COOKING TIME: 20 minutes
CALORIES: 350

INGREDIENTS FOR 3/4 SERVINGS

- 200 grams wholemeal flour

- 50 grams of oat flour

- 100 grams of black grapes

- 100 grams vegan raw cane sugar

- 1/2 teaspoon of cinnamon

- 80 grams of almond milk

- 60 ml sunflower oil

- ½ teaspoon cream of tartar (or baking powder)

DIRECTIONS

1. First, wash the grapes well and remove the grains.

2. Remove the seeds and cut them in half

3. In the meantime, in a large bowl put the wholemeal flour and the oat flour, the brown sugar, the cinnamon, the yeast and mix to mix the powders well.

4. Then add the liquids too.

5. Add the sunflower oil and almond milk.

6. Finally add the grapes that you have previously cut in half, eliminating the seeds if present.

7. Knead until the mixture is homogeneous and moist enough.

8. With the help of a spoon, take a quantity of dough about the size of a walnut, and place it on a baking sheet lined with parchment paper; there is no need to give it a shape.

9. Bake at 180 ° C for 20 minutes and after this time take the cookies out of the oven and let them cool completely on a wire rack.

10. You can serve them after they have cooled completely

Black grape and chocolate cookies

PREPARATION TIME: 20 minutes
COOKING TIME: 20 minutes
CALORIES: 389

INGREDIENTS FOR 3/4 SERVINGS

- 200 grams wholemeal flour
- 50 grams of sugar free cocoa flour
- 100 grams of white grapes
- 100 grams vegan raw cane sugar
- 1/2 teaspoon of vanilla powder
- 80 grams of rice milk
- 60 ml sunflower oil
- ½ teaspoon cream of tartar (or baking powder)
- 20 grams of dark chocolate vegan chips

DIRECTIONS

1. First, wash the white grapes well and remove the grains.
2. Remove the seeds and cut them in half
3. In the meantime, in a large bowl put the wholemeal flour and the cocoa powder, the brown sugar, the vanilla powder, the yeast and mix to mix the powders well.
4. Then add the liquids too.
5. Add the sunflower oil and rice milk.
6. Finally add the grapes (that you have previously cut in half) and chocolate vegan chips, eliminating the seeds if present.

7. Knead until the mixture is homogeneous and moist enough.

8. With the help of a spoon, take a quantity of dough about the size of a walnut, and place it on a baking sheet lined with parchment paper; there is no need to give it a shape.

9. Bake at 180 ° C for 20 minutes and after this time take the cookies out of the oven and let them cool completely on a wire rack.

10. You can serve them after they have cooled completely

Blueberries and vanilla cookies

PREPARATION TIME: 20 minutes
COOKING TIME: 20 minutes
CALORIES: 350

INGREDIENTS FOR 3/4 SERVINGS

- 200 grams wholemeal flour
- 50 grams of almond flour
- 100 grams of frozen blueberries
- 100 grams vegan raw cane sugar
- 1/2 teaspoon of vanilla powder
- 80 grams of almond milk
- 60 ml sunflower oil
- ½ teaspoon cream of tartar (or baking powder)

DIRECTIONS

1. First, take out blueberries from the freezer some hour before.
2. Wait until they will be defrost.
3. In the meantime, in a large bowl put the wholemeal flour and the almond flour, the brown sugar, the vanilla, the yeast and mix to mix the powders well.
4. Then add the liquids too.
5. Add the sunflower oil and almond milk.
6. Finally add the defrosted blueberries.
7. Knead until the mixture is homogeneous and moist enough.

8. With the help of a spoon, take a quantity of dough about the size of a walnut, and place it on a baking sheet lined with parchment paper; there is no need to give it a shape.

9. Bake at 180 ° C for 20 minutes and after this time take the cookies out of the oven and let them cool completely on a wire rack.

10. You can serve them after they have cooled completely

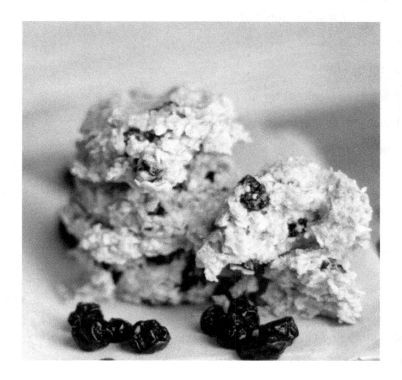

Apple and cinnamon cookies

PREPARATION TIME: 20 minutes
REST TIME: 30 minutes
COOKING TIME: 40 minutes
CALORIES: 270

INGREDIENTS FOR 4/5 SERVINGS

For the pastry:
- 250 grams wholemeal flour

- 80 ml corn oil

- 60 ml rice milk

- 8 grams of cream of tartar

- 110 grams of vegan whole cane sugar

For the filling:
- 2 apples

- 1 teaspoon of cinnamon powder

- 5 tablespoons of sugar

- 4 tablespoons of water

DIRECTIONS
1. First, prepare the cookie dough.

2. In a large bowl put the flour and baking powder and sift them to avoid lumps.

3. Blend the whole cane sugar in a mixer equipped with blades to pulverize it and avoid leaving grains inside the shortcrust pastry.

4. Add the powdered sugar to the flour.

5. Now pour the liquids, then the oil and rice milk and mix well, until you get a mixture that can be worked with your hands.

6. Transfer the mixture to a work surface and work it until you get a compact and homogeneous dough that you will wrap in cling film and let it rest in the refrigerator for 30 minutes.

7. In the meantime, prepare the filling with apples and cinnamon.

8. While the pastry rests, take the apples, wash them, peel them, cut them into small cubes, and put them in a saucepan together with the cinnamon and sugar, remembering to add 2 tablespoons of water.

9. Put on the heat and cook over medium-low heat for 20 minutes with the lid on, taking care to stir often and add a drop of water if necessary (it could be necessary to add two more tablespoons of water halfway through cooking).

10. After cooking, let it cool.

11. Meanwhile, take the pastry back and roll it out to a thickness of 3 millimetres.

12. If the dough releases oil, you can dab it with a paper towel and then proceed to spread it. It is a very crumbly pastry so, while you roll it out, be delicate.

13. Cut out the dough with a cookie cutter so that you always have an even number of discs.

14. Put a teaspoon of apple filling on the first disc and cover it with another disc, then gently press the edges with your fingers to seal the biscuit.

15. After preparing the apple and cinnamon biscuits, place them on a baking tray covered with parchment paper and bake (in a preheated oven) at 180 ° C for 20 minutes.

16. When they are cooked, take them out of the oven, let them cool and serve.

Pear and chocolate cookies

PREPARATION TIME: 20 minutes
REST TIME: 30 minutes
COOKING TIME: 40 minutes
CALORIES: 270

INGREDIENTS FOR 4/5 SERVINGS
For the pastry:
- 200 grams wholemeal flour

- 50 grams of sugar free cocoa

- 80 ml olive oil

- 60 ml coconut milk

- 8 grams of cream of tartar

- 110 grams of vegan whole cane sugar

For the filling:
- 2 pears

- 1 teaspoon of vanilla extract

- 5 tablespoons of sugar

- 4 tablespoons of water

DIRECTIONS
1. First, prepare the cookie dough.

2. In a large bowl put the flour, cocoa powder and baking powder and sift them to avoid lumps.

3. Blend the whole cane sugar in a mixer equipped with blades to pulverize it and avoid leaving grains inside the shortcrust pastry.

4. Add the powdered sugar to the flour.

5. Now pour the liquids, then the oil and coconut milk and mix well, until you get a mixture that can be worked with your hands.

6. Transfer the mixture to a work surface and work it until you get a compact and homogeneous dough that you will wrap in cling film and let it rest in the refrigerator for 30 minutes.

7. In the meantime, prepare the filling with pear and vanilla.

8. While the pastry rests, take the pears, wash them, peel them, cut them into small cubes, and put them in a saucepan together with the vanilla extract and sugar, remembering to add 2 tablespoons of water.

9. Put on the heat and cook over medium-low heat for 20 minutes with the lid on, taking care to stir often and add a drop of water if necessary (it could be necessary to add two more tablespoons of water halfway through cooking).

10. After cooking, let it cool.

11. Meanwhile, take the pastry back and roll it out to a thickness of 3 millimetres.

12. If the dough releases oil, you can dab it with a paper towel and then proceed to spread it. It is a very crumbly pastry so, while you roll it out, be delicate.

13. Cut out the dough with a cookie cutter so that you always have an even number of discs.

14. Put a teaspoon of pears filling on the first disc and cover it with another disc, then gently press the edges with your fingers to seal the biscuit.

15. After preparing the apple and cinnamon biscuits, place them on a baking tray covered with parchment paper and bake (in a preheated oven) at 180 ° C for 20 minutes.

16. When they are cooked, take them out of the oven, let them cool and serve.

Ginger and almond biscuits

PREPARATION TIME: 20 minutes
REST TIME: one night in the fridge
COOK TIME: 25 minutes
CALORIES: 90

INGREDIENTS FOR 3 SERVINGS

- 60 ml of water
- 5 grams of ginger
- 5 grams of cinnamon
- 55 grams of almond butter
- 70 grams of almond flour
- 80 grams of vegan cane sugar
- 25 grams of coconut flour
- 70 ml of almond milk
- Half a teaspoon of baking soda.

DIRECTIONS

1. Put the water and spices in a saucepan.
2. Stir often and as soon as it comes to a boil, remove from heat.
3. Add the almond butter and stir until completely melted.
4. Take a bowl, put the almond flour, coconut flour, brown sugar and baking soda inside and mix them together with a wooden spoon or spatula.
5. Now add the spice mixture and almond milk.
6. Knead the mixture with your hands until you have obtained a compact and lump-free dough.

7. Shape the dough into a ball, place it inside a sheet of cling film and let it rest in the fridge overnight.

8. After the standing time, preheat the oven to 150º C.

9. Divide the dough in half and roll out the first half on a pastry board with a rolling pin.

10. The dough must have a thickness of 3 millimetres.

11. Start cutting the dough with cookie cutters to your liking.

12. Repeat the operation with the other half and place the biscuits on a baking sheet covered with parchment paper.

13. Bake the biscuits for another 25-30 minutes.

14. Remove from the oven just a little and let them cool completely before serving.

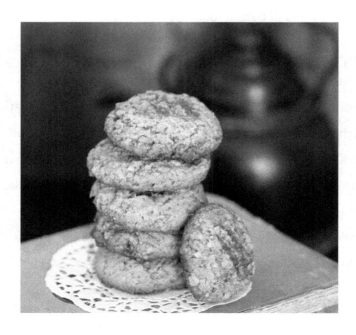

Spicy soy biscuits

PREPARATION TIME: 20 minutes
REST TIME: one night in the fridge
COOK TIME: 25 minutes
CALORIES: 90

INGREDIENTS FOR 3 SERVINGS

- 60 ml of water
- 5 grams of ginger
- 5 grams of cinnamon
- 1 pinch of nutmeg
- 55 grams of soy butter
- 70 grams of soy flour
- 80 grams of vegan cane sugar
- 25 grams of oat flour
- 70 ml of soymilk
- Half a teaspoon of baking soda.

DIRECTIONS

1. Put the water and spices in a saucepan.
2. Stir often and as soon as it comes to a boil, remove from heat.
3. Add the soy butter and stir until completely melted.
4. Take a bowl, put the oat flour, soy flour, brown sugar and baking soda inside and mix them together with a wooden spoon or spatula.
5. Now add the spice mixture and soymilk.
6. Knead the mixture with your hands until you have obtained a compact and lump-free dough.

7. Shape the dough into a ball, place it inside a sheet of cling film and let it rest in the fridge overnight.

8. After the standing time, preheat the oven to 175º C.

9. Divide the dough in half and roll out the first half on a pastry board with a rolling pin.

10. The dough must have a thickness of 3 millimeters.

11. Start cutting the dough with cookie cutters to your liking.

12. Repeat the operation with the other half and place the biscuits on a baking sheet covered with parchment paper.

13. Bake the biscuits for another 20 minutes.

14. Remove from the oven just a little and let them cool completely before serving.

Malt and chocolate cookies

PREPARATION TIME: 20 minutes
REST TIME: 30 minutes
CALORIES: 350

INGREDIENTS FOR 6 SERVINGS
- 150 grams of corn flour
- 100 grams of wholemeal flour
- 60 grams of malt
- 50 grams of vegan brown sugar
- 60 ml of olive oil
- 80 ml of soymilk
- 1 pinch of salt
- 1/2 teaspoon of cinnamon
- 2 g of cream of tartar
- 50 grams of vegan dark chocolate

DIRECTIONS
1. To begin, melt the dark chocolate in a double boiler and sift the flours.
2. On the other hand, dissolve the malt in the olive oil.
3. In a large bowl, mix all the dry ingredients (the two sifted flours, the vegan cane sugar) with the liquid ones (soymilk, malt dissolved in oil) until you get a smooth and soft mixture.
4. Let it rest for 30 minutes in the refrigerator covered with cling film.
5. At the end of the rest, roll out the pastry to a thickness of 5 mm and obtain, with the help of small pastry rings, some shapes for the biscuits.
6. Bake at 190 °C, static oven, for about 20 minutes.
7. When cookies are done, let cool and serve.

Chocolate and almonds sweet rectangles

PREPARATION TIME: 15 minutes
COOKING TIME: 20 minutes
CALORIES: 290

INGREDIENTS FOR 4 SERVINGS

- 100 grams of almond flour
- 6 tablespoons of sugar free cocoa powder
- 1 teaspoon of natural yeast powder
- 1/2 teaspoon of salt
- 150 ml of almond milk
- 50 grams of vegan cane sugar
- 1/2 teaspoon of vanillin

DIRECTIONS

1. First, preheat the oven to 180º C.

2. Grease a pan with a diameter of about 22 cm and line it with parchment paper.

3. As for the dough, beat the almond milk together with the vegan brown sugar in a bowl.

4. After they are blended you can put all the other ingredients together with them.

5. Mix and mix all the ingredients very well, then distribute the mixture obtained in the pan, levelling well.

6. Cook for about 15/20 minutes on the central rack (some ovens require more cooking time, so continue cooking until the crust solidifies, or place a toothpick to check the cooking in the centre of the cake).

7. Let the cake cool completely before serving.

8. Cut the cake into small rectangles and serve.

Chocolate and pistachios rectangles

PREPARATION TIME: 15 minutes
COOKING TIME: 20 minutes
CALORIES: 310

INGREDIENTS FOR 4 SERVINGS

- 100 grams of wholemeal flour

- 4 tablespoons of sugar free cocoa powder

- 2 tablespoons of finely chopped pistachios

- 1 teaspoon of natural yeast powder

- 1/2 teaspoon of salt

- 150 ml of rice milk

- 50 grams of vegan cane sugar

- 1/2 teaspoon of cinnamon

- Chopped pistachios (to decorate)

DIRECTIONS

1. First, peel and chop pistachios

2. Meanwhile, preheat the oven to 180º C.

3. Grease a pan with a diameter of about 22 cm and line it with parchment paper.

4. As for the dough, beat the rice milk together with the vegan brown sugar in a bowl.

5. After they are blended you can put all the other ingredients together with them.

6. Mix and mix all the ingredients very well, then distribute the mixture obtained in the pan, levelling well.

7. Cook for about 15/20 minutes on the central rack (some ovens require more cooking time, so continue cooking until the crust solidifies, or place a toothpick to check the cooking in the centre of the cake).

8. Let the cake cool completely before serving.

9. Cut the cake into small rectangles and serve with a topping of chopped pistachios.

Dates sweet ravioli

PREPARATION TIME: 40 minutes
COOKING TIME: 15 minutes
CALORIES: 510

INGREDIENTS FOR 4/5 SERVINGS

- 180 grams of wholemeal flour
- 50 ml of brown rice syrup
- 50 grams of sunflower oil
- 1 teaspoon of corn starch
- 30 ml of soymilk
- 1 pinch of vanilla powder
- 1 pinch of salt

For the dates stuffing:

- 50 grams of pitted dates
- 40 grams of dried red fruits
- 10 grams of walnuts
- 10 grams of almonds
- Juice of half a lemon
- ½ tablespoon of maple syrup
- ½ tablespoon of water
- 1 pinch of powdered ginger

DIRECTIONS

1. Start the recipe preparing the pastry.
2. Pour the wholemeal flour, corn starch, vanilla powder and a pinch of salt into a bowl and mix.

3. Add the sunflower oil, brown rice syrup and soymilk and knead everything until you get a soft but not sticky pastry.

4. Wrap the dough in plastic wrap and let it rest for an hour in the refrigerator.

5. Now prepare ravioli filling.

6. Blend the dates and red fruits in the food processor until you get a coarse mince. Then add the walnuts, almonds, ginger powder, lemon juice, maple syrup and water and blend until you get a sticky mixture that is still a little coarse.

7. After that, you can form sweet ravioli.

8. Roll out the pastry between two sheets of parchment paper with the help of a rolling pin until you get a very thin sheet (about 1 mm). With a sharp knife cut out squares of 9 cm per side and stuff each with a ball of filling slightly larger than a hazelnut.

9. Moisten the edges and fold the square in half to make a triangle. Seal the edges well, and then gently form a ravioli by matching the two vertices of the long side of the triangle together.

10. Place all the ravioli on a baking sheet lined with parchment paper and bake in a static oven at 180 ° C for 15 minutes.

11. Remove from the oven, let the cookies cool, and then transfer them to a wire rack to cool completely.

12. You can serve your sweet ravioli.

Apricot and almond sweet ravioli

PREPARATION TIME: 40 minutes
COOKING TIME: 15 minutes
CALORIES: 510

INGREDIENTS FOR 4/5 SERVINGS

- 180 grams of wholemeal flour
- 50 ml of brown rice syrup
- 50 grams of sunflower oil
- 1 teaspoon of corn starch
- 30 ml of soymilk
- 1 pinch of vanilla powder
- 1 pinch of salt

For the dates stuffing:

- 120 grams of apricots
- 30 grams of almonds
- Juice of half an orange
- ½ tablespoon of maple syrup
- ½ tablespoon of water
- 1 pinch of cinnamon

DIRECTIONS

1. Start the recipe preparing the pastry.
2. Pour the wholemeal flour, corn starch, vanilla powder and a pinch of salt into a bowl and mix.
3. Add the sunflower oil, brown rice syrup and soymilk and knead everything until you get a soft but not sticky pastry.

4. Wrap the dough in plastic wrap and let it rest for an hour in the refrigerator.

5. Now prepare ravioli apricot and almonds filling.

6. Blend the almonds, orange juice, cinnamon maple syrup and water and mix until you get a sticky mixture that is still a little coarse.

7. After that, you can form sweet ravioli.

8. Roll out the pastry between two sheets of parchment paper with the help of a rolling pin until you get a very thin sheet (about 1 mm). With a sharp knife cut out squares of 9 cm per side and stuff each with a ball of filling slightly larger than a hazelnut.

9. Moisten the edges and fold the square in half to make a triangle. Seal the edges well, and then gently form a ravioli by matching the two vertices of the long side of the triangle together.

10. Place all the ravioli on a baking sheet lined with parchment paper and bake in a static oven at 180 ° C for 15 minutes.

11. Remove from the oven, let the cookies cool, and then transfer them to a wire rack to cool completely.

12. You can serve your sweet ravioli.

Pistachio stuffed ravioli

PREPARATION TIME: 40 minutes
COOKING TIME: 15 minutes
CALORIES: 520

INGREDIENTS FOR 4/5 SERVINGS
- 160 grams of wholemeal flour
- 20 grams of almond flour
- 50 ml of brown rice syrup
- 50 grams of sunflower oil
- 1 teaspoon of corn starch
- 30 ml of almond milk
- 1 pinch of vanilla powder
- 1 pinch of salt

For the pistachio stuffing:
- 50 grams of chopped pistachios
- 4 tablespoons of homemade pistachio cream (see basic recipe)
- 10 grams of walnuts
- 10 grams of almonds
- ½ tablespoon of maple syrup
- ½ tablespoon of water

DIRECTIONS
1. Start the recipe preparing the pastry.
2. Pour the wholemeal flour, corn starch, almond flour, vanilla powder and a pinch of salt into a bowl and mix.
3. Add the sunflower oil, brown rice syrup and almond milk and knead everything until you get a soft but not sticky pastry.

4. Wrap the dough in plastic wrap and let it rest for an hour in the refrigerator.

5. Now prepare ravioli filling.

6. Blend the walnuts, almonds, pistachios, maple syrup, water, and pistachio cream and mix until you get a sticky mixture that is still a little coarse.

7. After that, you can form sweet ravioli.

8. Roll out the pastry between two sheets of parchment paper with the help of a rolling pin until you get a very thin sheet (about 1 mm). With a sharp knife cut out squares of 9 cm per side and stuff each with a ball of filling slightly larger than a hazelnut.

9. Moisten the edges and fold the square in half to make a triangle. Seal the edges well, and then gently form a ravioli by matching the two vertices of the long side of the triangle together.

10. Place all the ravioli on a baking sheet lined with parchment paper and bake in a static oven at 180 ° C for 15 minutes.

11. Remove from the oven, let the cookies cool, and then transfer them to a wire rack to cool completely.

12. You can serve your sweet ravioli.

Almond cream stuffed ravioli

PREPARATION TIME: 40 minutes
COOKING TIME: 15 minutes
CALORIES: 500

INGREDIENTS FOR 4/5 SERVINGS

- 180 grams of wholemeal flour

- 50 ml of brown rice syrup

- 50 grams of sunflower oil

- 1 teaspoon of corn starch

- 30 ml of almond milk

- 1 pinch of vanilla powder

- 1 pinch of salt

For the dates stuffing:

- 60 grams of almonds

- 10 grams of walnuts

- 50 grams of homemade almond cream (see basic recipe)

- 1 tablespoon of peanut butter

- ½ tablespoon of maple syrup

- ½ tablespoon of almond milk

- 1 pinch of vanilla powder

DIRECTIONS

1. Start the recipe preparing the pastry.

2. Pour the wholemeal flour, corn starch, vanilla powder and a pinch of salt into a bowl and mix.

3. Add the sunflower oil, brown rice syrup and soymilk and knead everything until you get a soft but not sticky pastry.

4. Wrap the dough in plastic wrap and let it rest for an hour in the refrigerator.

5. Now prepare almond cream ravioli filling.

6. Put in a mixer the walnuts, almonds, vanilla powder, peanut butter, almond cream maple syrup and almond milk and blend until you get a sticky mixture that is still a little coarse.

7. After that, you can form sweet ravioli.

8. Roll out the pastry between two sheets of parchment paper with the help of a rolling pin until you get a very thin sheet (about 1 mm). With a sharp knife cut out squares of 9 cm per side and stuff each with a ball of filling slightly larger than a hazelnut.

9. Moisten the edges and fold the square in half to make a triangle. Seal the edges well, and then gently form a ravioli by matching the two vertices of the long side of the triangle together.

10. Place all the ravioli on a baking sheet lined with parchment paper and bake in a static oven at 180 ° C for 15 minutes.

11. Remove from the oven, let the cookies cool, and then transfer them to a wire rack to cool completely.

12. You can serve your sweet ravioli.

Nutella and pistachios sweet ravioli

PREPARATION TIME: 40 minutes
COOKING TIME: 15 minutes
CALORIES: 500

INGREDIENTS FOR 4/5 SERVINGS
- 180 grams of wholemeal flour
- 50 ml of brown rice syrup
- 50 grams of sunflower oil
- 1 teaspoon of corn starch
- 30 ml of almond milk
- 1 pinch of vanilla powder
- 1 pinch of salt

For the dates stuffing:
- 60 grams of pistachios
- 10 grams of hazelnuts
- 50 grams of homemade Nutella cream (see basic recipe)
- ½ tablespoon of maple syrup
- ½ tablespoon of coconut milk
- 1 pinch of vanilla powder

DIRECTIONS
1. Start the recipe preparing the pastry.
2. Pour the wholemeal flour, corn starch, vanilla powder and a pinch of salt into a bowl and mix.
3. Add the sunflower oil, brown rice syrup and soymilk and knead everything until you get a soft but not sticky pastry.

4. Wrap the dough in plastic wrap and let it rest for an hour in the refrigerator.

5. Now prepare almond cream ravioli filling.

6. Put in a mixer the hazelnuts, pistachios, vanilla powder, Nutella cream, maple syrup and coconut milk and blend until you get a sticky mixture that is still a little coarse.

7. After that, you can form sweet ravioli.

8. Roll out the pastry between two sheets of parchment paper with the help of a rolling pin until you get a very thin sheet (about 1 mm). With a sharp knife cut out squares of 9 cm per side and stuff each with a ball of filling slightly larger than a hazelnut.

9. Moisten the edges and fold the square in half to make a triangle. Seal the edges well, and then gently form a ravioli by matching the two vertices of the long side of the triangle together.

10. Place all the ravioli on a baking sheet lined with parchment paper and bake in a static oven at 180 ° C for 15 minutes.

11. Remove from the oven, let the cookies cool, and then transfer them to a wire rack to cool completely.

12. You can serve your sweet ravioli.

Strawberry jam tart

PREPARATION TIME: 75 minutes
COOKING TIME: 150 minutes
CALORIES: 450

INGREDIENTS FOR 6/8 SERVINGS
- 100 grams wholemeal flour

- 150 grams spelt flour

- 80 grams of corn oil

- 60 ml of water

- 8 grams of natural yeast based on cream of tartar

- zest of 1/2 lemon

- 120 g of vegan whole cane sugar

For the strawberry homemade jam:
- 500 grams of strawberries

- 300 grams of vegan whole cane sugar

- 1/2 lemon juice

DIRECTIONS
1. First, prepare the homemade strawberry jam

2. Peel the fruit, taking care to wash it well under cold water and then remove the waste parts.

3. Cut the strawberries into small cubes of about 1 or 2 cm per side and put everything in a saucepan with high sides.

4. Cover the diced strawberries with whole sugar and let them rest for at least 10 minutes.

5. Add the lemon juice and cook over low heat for about 2 hours, stirring occasionally. If foam forms during cooking, take care to remove it with a skimmer.

6. The consistency that you will have to obtain at the end of cooking depends on the fruit chosen, but in general, the mixture must be thick and dense enough not to slip if placed on a smooth inclined saucer.

7. Now move on to the preparation of the pastry. In a large bowl put all the dry ingredients and sift them to avoid lumps. This step will make cooking easier and make the mixture more digestible. Blend the brown sugar in a blender equipped with blades in order to pulverize it and avoid leaving grains inside the shortcrust pastry.

8. Add the brown sugar and grated lemon zest to the flour. Add the powders to the liquids and mix well, until the mixture is workable with your hands. Transfer the mixture to a work surface, preferably a wooden one, and knead until a homogeneous dough is obtained.

9. Wrap the dough in cling film and let it rest in the refrigerator for at least 1 hour.

10. Once the rest period has passed, roll out the pastry on a work surface and then place it in the pan: it is a very crumbly pastry, so while you roll it out, be delicate.

11. Prick the bottom with the tines of a fork. With the leftover dough, make shapes to decorate the tart.

12. Now pour the jam into the raw shortcrust pastry shell and cook for 30/40 minutes at 180 C °, static oven.

13. Serve the tarts when it has cooled down

Berries homemade jam tart

PREPARATION TIME: 75 minutes
COOKING TIME: 150 minutes
CALORIES: 420

INGREDIENTS FOR 6/8 SERVINGS

- 250 grams wholemeal flour

- 80 grams of vegetal oil

- 60 ml of water

- 8 grams of natural yeast based on cream of tartar

- zest of 1/2 lime

- 120 g of vegan whole cane sugar

For the berries homemade jam:

- 500 grams of mixed berries

- 300 grams of vegan whole cane sugar

- 1/2 lime juice

DIRECTIONS

1. First, prepare the homemade jam.

2. Peel the berries fruit, taking care to wash it well under cold water and then remove the waste parts.

3. Cut the berries into small pieces and put everything in a saucepan with high sides.

4. Cover the diced berries with whole sugar and let them rest for at least 10 minutes.

5. Add the lime juice and cook over low heat for about 2 hours, stirring occasionally. If foam forms during cooking, take care to remove it with a skimmer.

6. The consistency that you will have to obtain at the end of cooking depends on the fruit chosen, but in general, the mixture must be thick and dense enough not to slip if placed on a smooth inclined saucer.

7. Now move on to the preparation of the pastry. In a large bowl put all the dry ingredients and sift them to avoid lumps. This step will make cooking easier and make the mixture more digestible. Blend the brown sugar in a blender equipped with blades in order to pulverize it and avoid leaving grains inside the shortcrust pastry.

8. Add the brown sugar and grated lime zest to the flour. Add the powders to the liquids and mix well, until the mixture is workable with your hands. Transfer the mixture to a work surface, preferably a wooden one, and knead until a homogeneous dough is obtained.

9. Wrap the dough in cling film and let it rest in the refrigerator for at least 1 hour.

10. Once the rest period has passed, roll out the pastry on a work surface and then place it in the pan: it is a very crumbly pastry, so while you roll it out, be delicate.

11. Prick the bottom with the tines of a fork. With the leftover dough, make shapes to decorate the tart.

12. Now pour the berries jam into the raw shortcrust pastry shell and cook for 30/40 minutes at 180 C °, static oven.

13. Serve the tarts when it has cooled down.

Apricot jam tart

PREPARATION TIME: 75 minutes
COOKING TIME: 150 minutes
CALORIES: 440

INGREDIENTS FOR 6/8 SERVINGS

- 150 grams wholemeal flour

- 100 grams spelt flour

- 80 grams of corn oil

- 60 ml of water

- 8 grams of natural yeast based on cream of tartar

- zest of 1/2 lemon

- 120 g of vegan whole cane sugar

- 500 grams of homemade apricot jam (see recipe)

DIRECTIONS

1. Start with the pastry preparation.

2. In a large bowl put all the dry ingredients and sift them to avoid lumps.

3. This step will make cooking easier and make the mixture more digestible. Blend the brown sugar in a blender equipped with blades in order to pulverize it and avoid leaving grains inside the shortcrust pastry.

4. Add the brown sugar and grated lemon zest to the flour. Add the powders to the liquids and mix well, until the mixture is workable with

your hands. Transfer the mixture to a work surface, preferably a wooden one, and knead until a homogeneous dough is obtained.

5. Wrap the dough in cling film and let it rest in the refrigerator for at least 1 hour.

6. Once the rest period has passed, roll out the pastry on a work surface and then place it in the pan: it is a very crumbly pastry, so while you roll it out, be delicate.

7. Prick the bottom with the tines of a fork. With the leftover dough, make shapes to decorate the tart.

8. Now pour the apricot jam into the raw shortcrust pastry shell and cook for 30/40 minutes at 180 C °, static oven.

9. Serve the tarts when it has cooled down.

Plant based drinks

Kiwi smoothie, almond milk and mint

PREPARATION TIME: 10 minutes
CALORIES: 176

INGREDIENTS FOR 4 PERSONS

- 500 grams of kiwi

- 500 ml of almond milk

- 2 tablespoons of vegan brown sugar

- 1 tablespoon of homemade mint syrup

- Mint leaves to decorate

DIRECTIONS

1. Peel and wash the kiwis, then cut them into small pieces.

2. Put the kiwi in the blender glass with the milk, mint syrup and sugar.

3. Blend on high speed until you get a thick and creamy smoothie.

4. Now put the smoothie in the glasses.

5. Decorate with mint leaves and serve.

Honey lemonade

PREPARATION TIME: 5 minutes
CALORIES: 77

INGREDIENTS FOR 4 SERVINGS
- 6 lemons
- 800 ml of water
- 2 tablespoons of honey
- 10 ice cubes
- 4 slices of lemon

DIRECTIONS
1. Squeeze the lemons and strain the juice into a jug.
2. Now add the honey and mix well, until the honey is well incorporated.
3. Pour in the water and mix again.
4. Put the lemonade to cool in the fridge.
5. When it is time to serve it, add the lemon slices and ice and serve in glasses with straws.

Peach, strawberry and lemon extract

PREPARATION TIME: 5 minutes
CALORIES: 76

INGREDIENTS FOR 4 SERVINGS

- 5 peaches

- 300 grams of strawberries

- Half a lemon

DIRECTIONS

1. Peel the peaches and wash them. Cut them in half, remove the stone, and then cut them into pieces.

2. Wash the strawberries and then cut them in half.

3. Peel the lemon.

4. Put peach, lemon and strawberries in the extractor and pour the juice into the glasses.

5. Served with ice and straws.

Mango and nut smoothie

PREPARATION TIME: 10 minutes
CALORIES: 272

INGREDIENTS FOR 4 SERVINGS

- 4 mangoes
- 16 shelled walnuts
- 2 lemons
- 400 ml of almond milk
- 2 teaspoons of honey
- 12 ice cubes

DIRECTIONS

1. Peel the mangoes, wash them, cut them first in half and then into small pieces.
2. Put the mango pulp in the glass of the blender together with the walnuts, the honey and the almond milk and the filtered juice of the lemons.
3. Turn on the blender and blend at maximum speed for 1 minute.
4. Now add the ice cubes and blend again, until you get a thick and creamy mixture.
5. Pour into glasses, add straws and serve.

Smoothie with strawberries, banana and nuts

PREPARATION TIME: 10 minutes
CALORIES: 230

INGREDIENTS FOR 4 SERVINGS

- 4 bananas
- 12 shelled walnuts
- 32 strawberries
- 400 ml of coconut milk
- 8 ice cubes

DIRECTIONS

1. Peel the bananas and then cut them into small pieces.
2. Wash the strawberries and then cut them in half.
3. Put the walnuts, strawberries and bananas in the blender glass.
4. Add the coconut milk and blend on high speed for one minute.
5. Now add the ice cubes and blend until you have a smooth and homogeneous mixture.
6. Put the smoothie in the glasses and serve.

Smoothie of apple, kiwi and black grapes

PREPARATION TIME: 10 minutes
CALORIES: 126

INGREDIENTS FOR 4 SERVINGS

- 2 apples
- 3 kiwis
- a bunch of black grapes
- 12 strawberries
- 1 lemon
- 12 ice cubes
- 200 ml of unsweetened orange juice

DIRECTIONS

1. Peel the kiwi, wash them and then cut them into pieces.
2. Wash the strawberries and then cut them in half.
3. Wash the grapes, cut them in half and remove the seeds.
4. Peel the kiwi, wash them and then cut them into pieces.
5. Wash the strawberries and then cut them in half.
6. Wash the grapes, cut them in half and remove the seeds.
7. Peel the apples, wash them, cut them in half and remove the seeds.
8. Put the kiwi, apples, strawberries and grapes in the blender glass.
9. Wash the lemon, grate the zest and strain the juice in a blender.
10. Add the orange juice and ice cubes and blend until you get a smooth and homogeneous mixture.
11. Put the smoothie in the glasses, sprinkle with the grated lemon zest, the straws and serve.

PREPARATION TIME: 10 minutes
CALORIES: 138

INGREDIENTS FOR 4 SERVINGS

- 450 grams of peaches
- 200 grams of soy yogurt
- 200 ml of almond milk
- 80 grams of dates
- 1 tablespoon of honey
- 1 tablespoon of vanilla extract
- 12 ice cubes

DIRECTIONS

1. Peel the peaches, wash them, remove the stone and then cut them into pieces.
2. Cut the dates into small pieces.
3. Put the peaches and dates in the blender glass.
4. Add honey, yogurt, almond milk and vanilla extract.
5. Blend at high speed for one minute.
6. Now add the ice and blend again for another minute.
7. Now put the milkshake in the glasses, add the straws and serve.

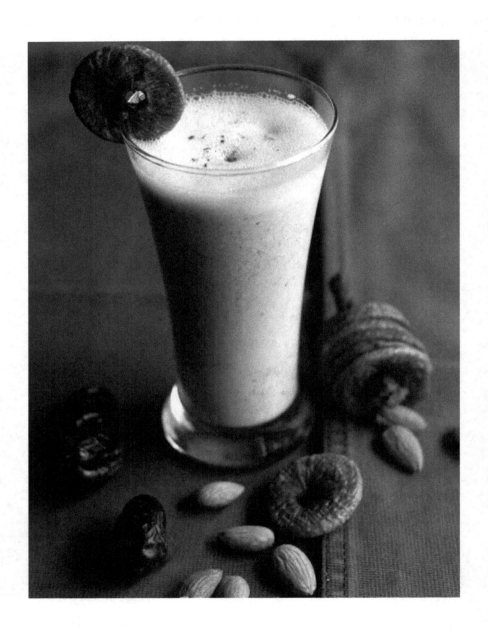

CPSIA information can be obtained
at www.ICGtesting.com
Printed in the USA
BVHW041416180621
609826BV00004B/857